Contents

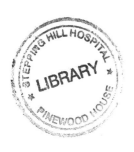

Preface

This book is intended for use by all personnel involved in the ECG monitoring of the patient with a dysrhythmia, chest pain, or is otherwise acutely ill. Whether ambulance personnel involved in the patient's pre-hospital care or nurses, junior medical or other staff involved in the in-hospital phase of patient care.

My thanks go to my colleagues in Gloucestershire who helped in the original assessment and writing of this book [1981] and to Dawn, my friend and colleague in Resuscitation, for more recent support.

2005

J. GARDINER
Hereford

Introduction: What is an ECG?

An electrocardiogram (ECG) is a recording of the electrical activity of the heart, throughout the cardiac cycle (both normal and abnormal). Electrodes placed on the patient's skin pick up the activity. The resultant ECG is amplified and may be displayed either on a screen or on paper. The electrodes on the skin pick up a wave of activity or *depolarization* moving along each cell, within the heart. This wave of depolarization causes contraction of the affected part. After contraction the muscle cell returns to its resting state, in other words it *repolarizes*. The skin electrodes may also pick up this activity. If the wave of depolarization moves towards the electrode it will result in a positive or upward deflection on the ECG. If the wave of depolarization moves away from the electrode the result is a negative or downward deflection of the ECG.

If the position of the electrode receiving the electrical impulses is varied the resultant deflections on the ECG may vary in pattern (figure 1).

Figure 1 The effect of depolarization on the ECG.

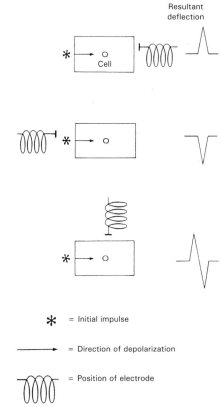

1

The heart

The heart is a muscular pump which pumps deoxygenated blood from the body to the lungs, and oxygenated blood, from the lungs to the body. For this action to take place the heart is made up of two completely separate halves, each half consisting of a receiving chamber (*atrium*) and a pumping chamber (*ventricle*). There is a valve that prevents the back flow of the blood at the exit of each chamber. The muscle (*myocardium*) in the walls of each chamber is thinnest in the atria, which only have to pump blood into the ventricles, thicker in the right ventricle, which pumps the blood into the lungs, and thickest in the left ventricle which pumps the blood throughout the body. On the inner surface of the myocardium is the *endocardium*, a smooth lining, and outside is the tough protective *pericardium* (figure 2).

The conduction pathway

All cells within the heart can originate their own electrical activity which is

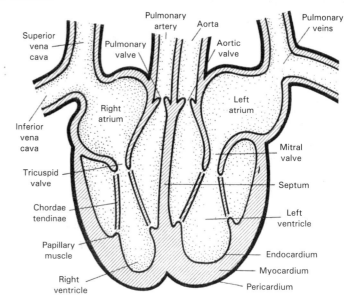

Figure 2. The heart

then transmitted along a conduction 'pathway' of specialized cells (figure 3). The pathway consists of: the *sinoatrial (S-A) node*, a collection of cells situated in the wall of the right atrium near the entrance of the superior vena cava.

Here depolarization is initiated at a rate of approximately 80 beats per minute. The rate is affected by the autonomic nervous system (the parasympathetic slows the rate and the sympathetic increases the rate), and also by the effect of some hormones. The impulse from the S-A node spreads across the atria causing a wave

Figure 3. The electrical conduction pathway of the heart

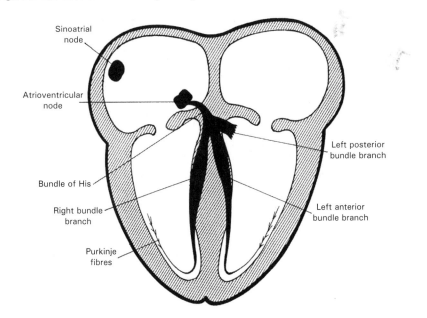

Sinoatrial node

Atrioventricular node

Bundle of His

Right bundle branch

Purkinje fibres

Left posterior bundle branch

Left anterior bundle branch

of depolarization that results in atrial contraction. The impulses then reach and pause at the *atrioventricular (A-V) node*. This is also a collection of specialized cells situated just to the right of the interatrial septum (near the coronary sinus).

After a slight pause the impulse is allowed to pass on. If for some reason the S-A node is unable to initiate any impulses the A-V node may do this but at a slower rate of approximately 60 beats per minute (normally the faster rate from the S-A node controls the heart). Running from the A-V node into the posterior part of the interventricular septum is the electrical connection between the atria and the ventricles, *the bundle of His*. This is approximately 22 mm long and divides into its right bundle branch (to the right ventricle), and a much thicker left bundle branch. The latter divides almost immediately into an anterior branch (supplying the anterior part of the septum and left ventricle) and a posterior branch (supplying the posterior part of the septum and the posterior and inferior parts of the left ventricle).

Both branches end as numerous fine fibres running into the ventricular myocardium, known as *Purkinje fibres*. The impulse passed on from the A-V node passes very quickly along the bundle of His, bundle branches and Purkinje fibres, resulting in ventricular depolarization and contraction. In some circumstances impulses may originate in the Purkinje fibres (although at a rate of only 40 beats per minute or less). During ventricular depolarization the atria repolarize (return to the previous resting state). After their depolarization the ventricles repolarize before the cycle starts again.

The normal ECG waveform

The normal waveform seen may vary depending upon the exact location of the skin electrodes. There are twelve different views normally used for diagnostic purposes – the twelve-lead ECG.

For monitoring purposes, one of three leads or views are used – leads II, III or VI – these are positive leads, the waveforms are mainly above the isoelectric line. All descriptions given are of the rhythm seen via lead II (figure 4).

The various waves seen on the ECG are labelled with letters to aid description – P, Q, R, S, T, U. The first wave seen is the P wave. This is normally a positive (upright) deflection and is caused by atrial depolarization. After a slight pause the next three waves (Q, R, S) appear very close to each other and together represent ventricular depolarization. Often the waves are all present, but even if they are not (and this may be quite normal) the complex is known as a *QRS complex*.

Figure 4. The progress of depolarization (lead II)

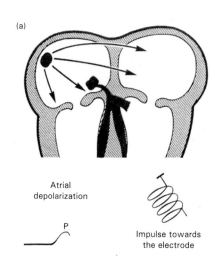

(a)

Atrial depolarization

P

Impulse towards the electrode

(b)

Delay/pause at the atrioventricular node

P

The *Q wave* may not be seen at all and when it is, is frequently very small. This is a negative deflection, and is followed by a positive deflection, often quite large, and known as the *R wave*. The negative wave seen after the R wave is the *S wave*. As mentioned above an *R wave* only, or a QR or an RS wave, etc. may be present.

After a pause the QRS complex is followed by another positive wave, the *T wave* representing ventricular repolarization. Occasionally another small positive wave may be seen after the T wave, known as the *U wave*.

There are many differences of opinion over what exactly is the significance of the U wave. When seen on a single monitoring lead it must be correctly observed as a U wave and not an extra P wave (when seen the U

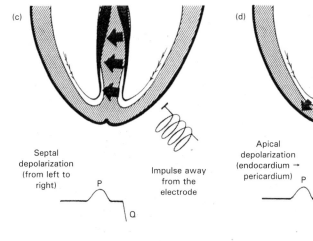

(c) Septal depolarization (from left to right)

Impulse away from the electrode

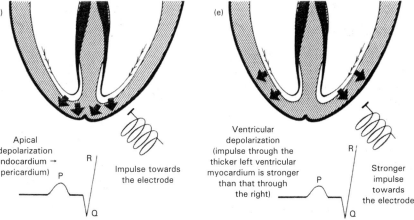

(d) Apical depolarization (endocardium → pericardium)

Impulse towards the electrode

(e) Ventricular depolarization (impulse through the thicker left ventricular myocardium is stronger than that through the right)

Stronger impulse towards the electrode

wave is usually quite different from the P wave).

The pause between the P wave and the QRS complex (the pause of the impulse at the A-V node) is normally isoelectric (flat), and the distance from the beginning of the P wave to the beginning of the QRS complex is known as the *P–R interval*. The pause between the QRS complex and the T wave (between the end of ventricular depolarization and start of ventricular repolarization) is normally isoelectric, and known as the *S-T segment*.

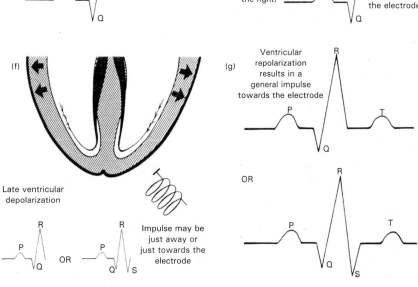

(f) Late ventricular depolarization

Impulse may be just away or just towards the electrode

(g) Ventricular repolarization results in a general impulse towards the electrode

OR

Timing

The ECG seen on the monitor or paper strip can be recorded at various rates, although normally the rate is 25 mm/ sec.

There are both vertical and horizontal lines on the paper. The horizontal lines indicate voltage of the waveform and are normally standardized at 10 mm (two large squares) equalling 1 millivolt (mV). The vertical lines indicate time, at a rate of 25 mm/sec, each large square (5 mm) is equal to 0.2 sec, and each small square (1 mm) is equal to 0.04 sec. These can be used in the estimation of intervals in the ECG and the atrial and/or ventricular rate (figure 5).

Figure 5(a). Normal range of intervals on the ECG

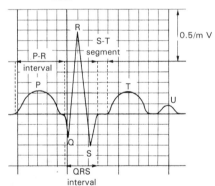

P–R interval adult – 0.18–0.2 sec
child – 0.15–0.18 sec

QRS interval – 0.07–0.1 sec

Figure 5(b). Calculation of rate
(Only accurate if the rhythm is regular.)
(i) Count the number of QRS complexes in a three second period (15 large squares) and multiply by 20.

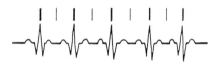

(ii) Find an R wave (or similar obvious wave, such as S) on a thick vertical line: divide the number of large squares between that R wave and the same wave on the next complex into 300. For example (above)

300/2 = 150 bpm.

(iii) As (ii) but divide the number of small squares between complexes into 1500. For example,

1500/10 = 150 bpm.

Sinus rhythm

Description

Normal rhythm, with the impulse originating in the sinoatrial node, and following a normal pathway (figure 6).

ECG characteristics

- Rate: 60-100 bpm
- Rhythm: regular
- P waves: normal, preceding each QRS complex
- P–R interval: normal (0.16–0.2 sec)
- QRS complex: normal

Clinical significance

Nil, is a normal rhythm, therefore no treatment is required.

Figure 6. Sinus Rhythm

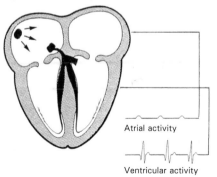

Atrial activity

Ventricular activity

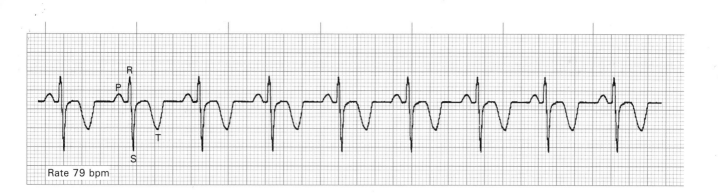

Rate 79 bpm

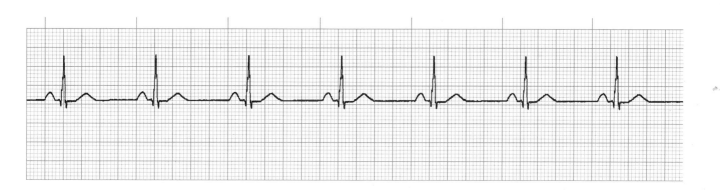

Sinus dysrhythmias

Sinus bradycardia

Description

Impulse originates in the sinoatrial node (figure 7).

ECG characteristics

- Rate: below 60 bpm
- Rhythm: regular
- P waves: normal, preceding each QRS complex
- P–R interval: normal
- QRS complex: normal

Clinical significance

May be normal in athletic young adults, or may be due to increased parasympathetic tone (vagus nerve), damage to S-A node, hypoxia or excess of cardiac drugs (such as *digoxin, β blockers,* etc.).

The slow rate may result in a reduction in the blood pressure and deterioration in tissue perfusion.

Treatment

No treatment is required if the blood pressure is maintained and the patient is not compromised. However, treatment may be required if:

(1) Blood pressure is significantly low (systolic < 90 mm Hg).
(2) Heart rate is < 40 bpm.
(3) There is evidence of heart failure.
(4) Ventricular arrhythmias appear.

The drug of choice is *atropine* in a dose of 500 mcg i.v. repeated as required to a maximum of 3 mg.

The patient should also be placed flat to assist the cerebral circulation, and high flow oxygen therapy given to reduce the risk of cerebral hypoxia (which may be causing the bradycardia). Also relate to current Resuscitation Council (UK) guidelines on the management of Bradycardia.

Figure 7. Sinus bradycardia

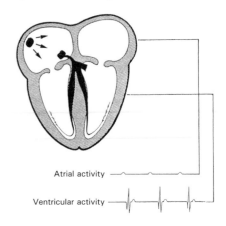

Atrial activity

Ventricular activity

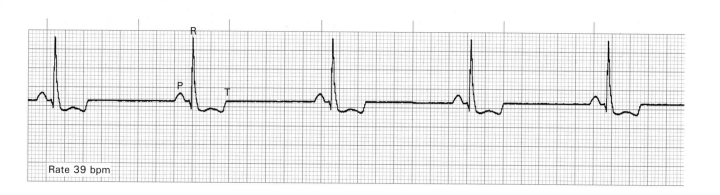

Rate 39 bpm

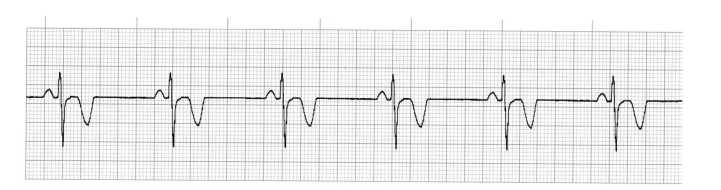

Sinus tachycardia

Description

Impulse originates in the sinoatrial node (figure 8).

ECG characteristics

- Rate: 100–180 bpm
- Rhythm: regular
- P waves: normal, if the rate is very fast the P wave may be buried in the T wave of the previous beat
- P–R interval: normal
- QRS complex: normal

Clinical significance

May be due to increased sympathetic stimulation caused by pain, fever or anxiety, or may be the normal reaction to exercise. It may also be due to haemorrhage, early hypoxia, congestive cardiac failure, left ventricular failure, or as a reaction to some drugs that are used to treat bradycardia such as *atropine or adrenaline*.

If the rate is not too high there may be little effect on the patient. If over 120–140 bpm the cardiac output may be reduced due to decreased ventricular filling time. This may result in a lowered blood pressure, reduced tissue perfusion and its associated signs and symptoms.

The increased cardiac workload, but decreased coronary supply to the myocardium, may result in myocardial ischaemia and the possibility of chest pain.

Treatment

Relieve pain if present by appropriate analgesia, reassure the patient, relieve anxiety, relieve hypoxia with oxygen therapy, control haemorrhage, treat heart failure, if present.

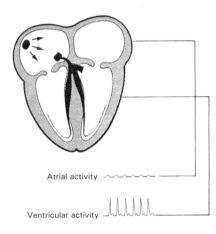

Figure 8. Sinus tachycardia

Atrial activity

Ventricular activity

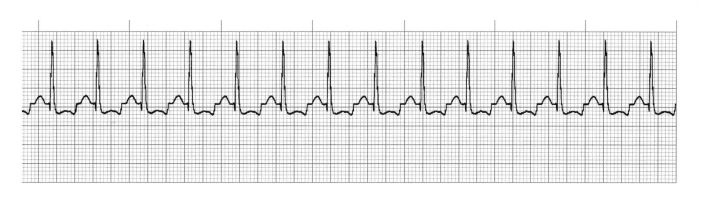

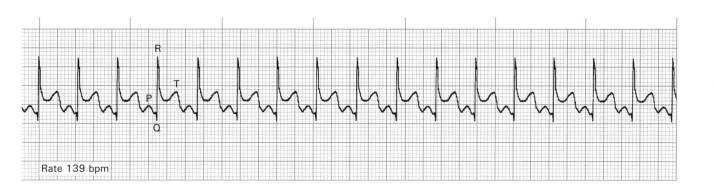

Rate 139 bpm

11

Sinus arrhythmia

Description

Impulse originates in the sinoatrial node, but the rate at which the impulses appear varies. If the patient's respiratory rate is observed, note that the heart rate increases during inspiration and decreases during expiration (figure 9).

ECG characteristics

- Rate: variable (but normally between 60–100 bpm)
- Rhythm: irregular (but regularly irregular in relation to respiration)
- P waves: normal
- P–R interval: normal
- QRS complex: normal

Clinical significance

This is accepted as a normal phenomenon in young people, when caused by variations in the parasympathetic activity on the sinoatrial node during respiration. An uncommon form of sinus arrhythmia which occurs without any apparent relationship to respiration or external factors may be indicative of heart disease.

Treatment

As this is a normal phenomenon no treatment is required.

Figure 9. Sinus arrhythmia

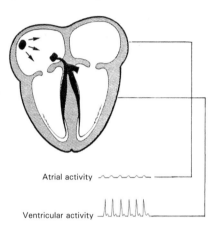

Atrial activity

Ventricular activity

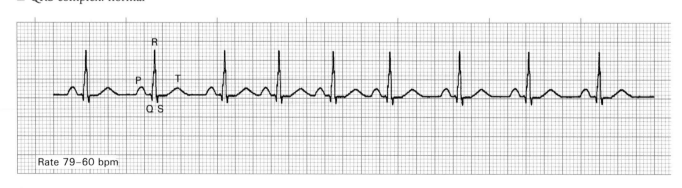

Rate 79–60 bpm

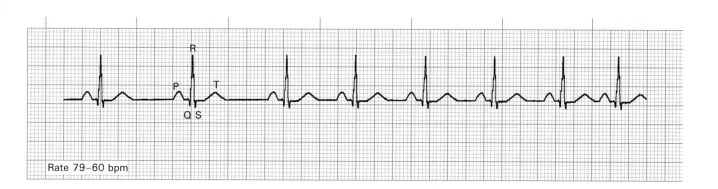

Rate 79–60 bpm

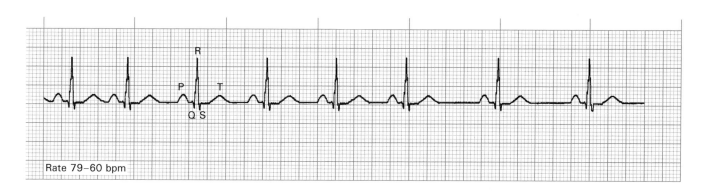

Rate 79–60 bpm

Sinus arrest

Description

The impulse originates in the sinoatrial node, resulting in a sinus rhythm or sinus bradycardia. There is a pause in the rhythm due to a failure of the S-A node to originate an impulse, and this results in a completely missed beat, following which the previous rhythm may be recommenced. There may be other periods of sinus arrest (figure 10). The distance between the R wave prior to the sinus arrest and the R wave after may or may not be double the normal R-R interval.

Occasionally another ectopic focus in the heart (atria, A-V node or ventricles) may appear during the pause as an escape beat. Note that the distance between the R wave prior to the sinus arrest and the R wave of the escape beat is greater than the normal R-R interval. The P wave of the escape beat (if present) may be abnormal, the QRS complex may or may not be normal depending upon the origin of the escape beat. The R-R interval from the escape beat to the next normal beat may be normal or slightly greater than normal.

ECG characteristics

- Rate: normal (60–100 bpm) or slow
- Rhythm: normal except for the pause left by the missed beat
- P waves: absent during sinus arrest otherwise normal (may be abnormal or absent if escape beat is present)
- P–R interval: absent during sinus arrest, otherwise normal
- QRS complex: absent during sinus arrest, otherwise normal (may or may not be normal if escape beat is present)

Clinical significance

If rate is otherwise normal the patient will be unaffected. The cause may be increased parasympathetic activity, it may be drug-induced (such as through an excess of digoxin) or appear as a result of ischaemic heart disease. If the overall heart rate is low the patient may suffer the effects of a lowered cardiac output, and will need to be treated to relieve the symptoms of the lowered cardiac output (see sinus bradycardia). If caused by digoxin excess the drug may be withheld until the blood level is lower.

Figure 10. Sinus arrest

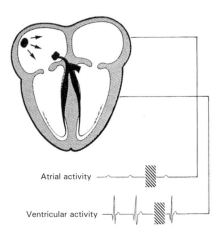

Atrial activity

Ventricular activity

Period of arrest

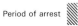

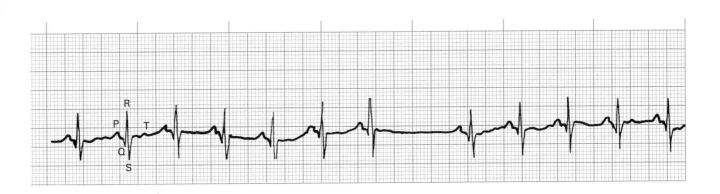

Supraventricular dysrhythmias

Wandering atrial pacemaker

Description

The impulses may originate in the S-A node, anywhere in the atria or in the A-V node. The site of impulse continually changes, resulting in varying shapes and sizes of the P wave, the QRS will remain normal (figure 11).

ECG characteristics

- Rate: normal
- Rhythm: slightly irregular (may appear regular)
- P waves: vary in size and shape depending on the exact origin of the impulse
- P–R interval: varies depending upon site of impulse (from 0.2 sec at the S-A node to 0.12 sec at the A-V node)
- QRS complex: normal

Clinical significance

May be a relatively normal phenomenon caused by increased parasympathetic stimulation, excessive digoxin or ischaemic heart disease. It does not usually affect the patient, although it may be a warning of other atrial dysrhythmias.

Treatment

If the rhythm has no adverse effect on the patient then no treatment is required, although the digoxin therapy may need to be altered if this is the cause of the dysrhythmia.

Figure 11. Wandering atrial pacemaker

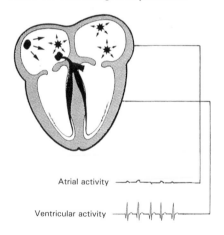

Atrial activity

Ventricular activity

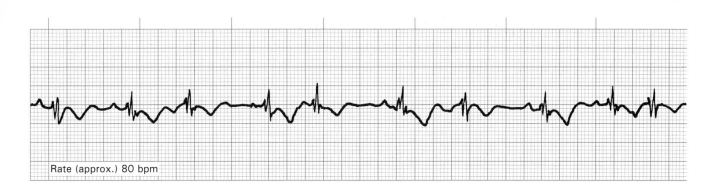

Rate (approx.) 80 bpm

Premature atrial contractions (atrial ectopics)

Description

A premature beat arises from an ectopic focus, which originates an impulse, before the next normal beat is due. Therefore in an otherwise 'normal' rhythm an ectopic beat appears. The R-R interval between the ectopic beat and the previous normal beat will be less than the normal R-R interval. The R-R interval between the ectopic beat and the following normal beat may be longer than the normal R-R interval. The pause after the ectopic beat, and before the next normal beat, is known as a *compensatory pause*. After the atrial ectopic the rhythm returns to normal until the next ectopic beat (figure 12).

ECG characteristics

- Rate: normal
- Rhythm: regular except for the atrial ectopics
- P waves: normal, but abnormal prior to the atrial ectopics
- P–R interval: normal, except that of the atrial ectopic and then will vary depending upon the site of the ectopic focus.
- QRS complex: normal

Clinical significance

Premature atrial contractions may be a normal phenomenon and may be caused by emotional disturbances or the use of tobacco, tea or coffee. They may also be due to digoxin toxicity or to organic heart disease causing damage to the atrial. The presence of atrial ectopics (if very frequent) may be a warning of other atrial dysrhythmias.

Treatment

Usually no treatment required unless:
(1) The dysrhythmia is due to digoxin toxicity, assess blood level and alter the regime.
(2) The dysrhythmia is due to atrial damage/heart failure, in which case appropriate anti-dysrhythmics may be prescribed.

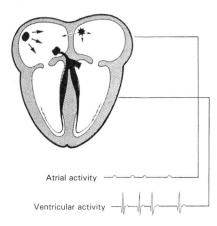

Figure 12. **Premature atrial contractions**

Atrial activity

Ventricular activity

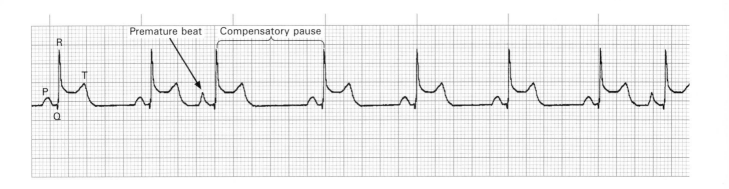

Premature beat Compensatory pause

R

T

P

Q

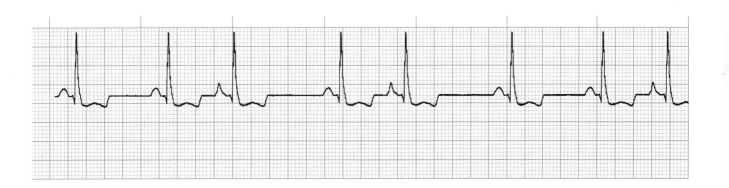

Atrial flutter

Description

The impulses originate within the atria. Either one or several ectopic foci initiate impulses very rapidly (at a rate of 220–350 times per minute). There is also a theory of a circular movement of impulses within the atria with the same effect. The rapid atrial rate gives rise to a sawtooth appearance on the ECG (known as F waves).

The ventricles are unable to respond to such a rapid rate, so the A-V node blocks many of the impulses resulting in more F waves than QRS complexes (figure 13).

ECG characteristics

- Rate: atrial rate 220–350/min.
- Ventricular rate varies with degree of block at the A-V node, which may be 60–180 bpm
- Rhythm: Atrial rhythm is regular.
- Ventricular rhythm often regular but may be irregular if the degree of block varies
- P waves: None seen – instead the characteristic sawtooth flutter waves
- P–R interval: difficult to determine, F–R interval may be apparently normal on the complexes conducted through the A-V node
- QRS complex: normal

Clinical significance

If the ventricular rate is normal there may be little adverse effect on the patient. If the ventricular rate is rapid, >140/min, there may be some loss in cardiac output, resulting in a lowered blood pressure, reduced tissue perfusion and associated signs and symptoms, due to reduced ventricular filling time. There may be some chest pain due to increased ventricular workload and decreased coronary artery flow (decreased oxygen supply to the myocardium).

The dysrhythmia may occur because of organic heart disease, damage to the atria, congestive cardiac failure or increased sympathetic tone. If due to disease, such as rheumatic heart disease or thyrotoxicosis, the arrhythmia may progress to atrial fibrillation.

Treatment

If the ventricular rate is normal the patient may be unaffected, but if it is rapid the patient may show the signs and symptoms of a lowered cardiac output.

Initially the treatment will be supportive – patient at rest (in most comfortable position) – upright if dyspnoeic, flat if hypotensive. Oxygen therapy is given. The patient can then be treated with antidysrhythmics *or cardioversion* (synchronised DC shock), together with the treatment of any associated disease. Also relate to current Resuscitation Council (UK) guidelines on the management of Atrial Fibrillation.

Figure 13. Atrial flutter.

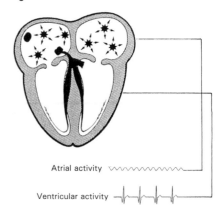

Atrial activity

Ventricular activity

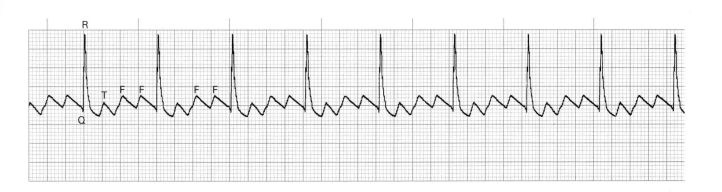

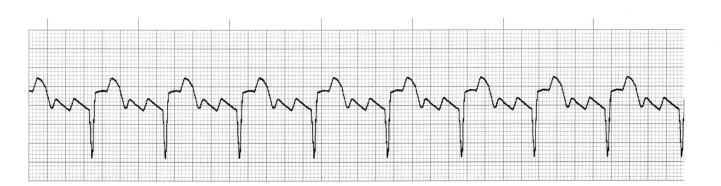

Atrial fibrillation

Description

Similar to that of atrial flutter, but there are usually more atrial ectopic foci and the atrial rate is in excess of 360 bpm, resulting in a completely uncoordinated twitching of the atria. There is a very variable rate of block at the A-V node resulting in a totally irregular response by the ventricular myocardium, so the ventricular rate is very irregular (irregularly irregular) and between 60–160 bpm. Because of the rate and irregularity some of the beats are poor in volume and may not be felt at the radial pulse (the difference in heart rate and radial pulse rate is the *pulse deficit*). The fibrillation waves seen on the ECG may vary in amplitude and may be either coarse or fine in appearance (figure 14).

ECG characteristics

- Rate: atrial rate >360/min; ventricular rate 60–150/min
- Rhythm: totally irregular
- P waves: none seen, only small irregular F waves
- P–R interval: not identifiable
- QRS complexes: normal

Clinical significance

May be due to increased sympathetic tone, damage to the atria due to organic heart disease, congestive cardiac failure or associated with mitral valve disease.
If the ventricular rate is rapid there may be a lowering of cardiac output, as with atrial flutter.

Treatment

See atrial flutter (page 20).

Atrial flutter/ fibrillation

Occasionally the ECG will show a combination of atrial flutter and atrial fibrillation on the same trace. This may be termed a *flutter/fibrillation*.

Figure 14. Atrial fibrillation

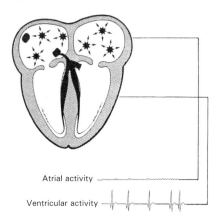

Atrial activity

Ventricular activity

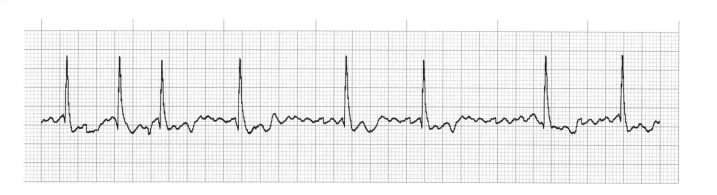

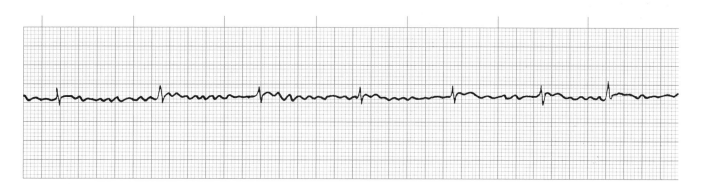

Junctional (nodal) rhythm

Description

If the impulse should originate from within the A-V node, either as an ectopic beat, escape beat or a complete rhythm, it is termed a junctional or nodal ectopic, beat or rhythm. The impulse originating in the region of the A-V node travels both up into the atria (retrograde conduction) and down into the ventricles.

If the S-A node does not function the A-V node may take over as the pacemaker of the heart. The ventricular rate then being approximately 40–65 bpm. The rhythm may be temporary or permanent, and the rate may increase up to 200 bpm if a tachycardia is present (figure 15).

There are three main areas from which the impulse may arise:
(1) Just above the A-V node (high nodal),
(2) Within the A-V node (mid-nodal), or
(3) Just below the A-V node (low

nodal), all resulting in a slight difference on the ECG.

High nodal
The impulse has time to activate the atria before the A-V node allows the impulse to pass on to the ventricles, so an inverted P wave is seen prior to the QRS complex.

Mid-nodal
The impulse reaches the atria at the same time as it reaches the ventricles, so no P wave is seen prior to the QRS complex, but the P wave may be seen as a notch on the QRS complex.

Low nodal
The impulse reaches the ventricles before the A-V node allows the impulse to pass on to the atria, so the P wave (inverted) is seen *after* the QRS complex but *before* the T wave.

All three types are generally classed together as junctional or nodal.

ECG characteristics

- Rate: normal 40–65/min (rarely up to 200/min)
- Rhythm: regular
- P waves: may be inverted prior to the complex, lost in the complex or inverted after the complex
- P–R interval: variable or absent
- QRS complex: normal but may be distorted if the P wave is buried in the complex (mid-nodal)

Clinical significance

The dysrhythmia may be due to damage to the A-V node in ischaemic heart disease, increased sympathetic activity (tachycardia), increased parasympathetic activity (bradycardia), congestive cardiac failure, hypoxia or overdose of some cardiac drugs.

If only the occasional nodal ectopic is noted there are unlikely to be any ill effects. If there is a very slow or very fast ventricular rate there may be some loss of cardiac output, resulting in hypotension, reduced tissue perfusion (pale, cold, clammy skin) and, if a fast rate, chest pain.

Treatment

If there is no adverse effect on the patient then no treatment is required. If the dysrhythmia results in a lowering of cardiac output supportive treatment will be required (including oxygen therapy, etc.). If the rate is slow atropine 500 mcg i.v, repeated, as required, up to a maximum of 3 mg may be administered, or external pacing prior to invasive pacing may be necessary (see sinus bradycardia).

If the rate is rapid, vagal stimulation and the use of anti-dysrhythmics or cardioversion may be required (see Supraventricular tachycardia page 28).

Figure 15. Junctional (nodal) arrhythmias

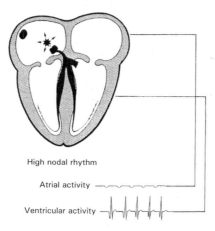

High nodal rhythm

Atrial activity

Ventricular activity

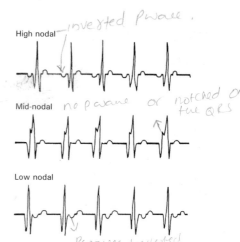

High nodal — *inverted P wave.*

Mid-nodal — *no p wave or notched on the QRS*

Low nodal — *P wave inverted*

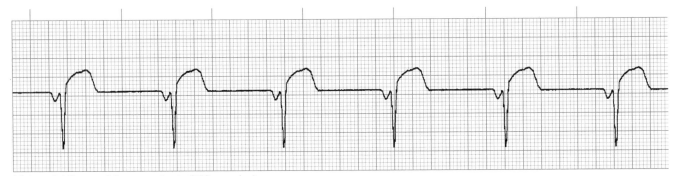

High nodal (inverted P wave prior to QRS complex)

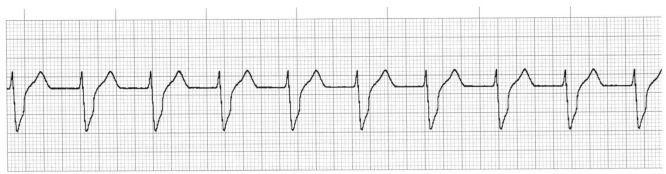

Mid-nodal (inverted P wave as a notch on the QRS complex)

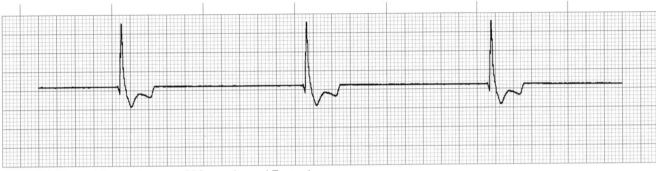

Low nodal (inverted P wave between QRS complex and T wave)

Paroxysmal atrial tachycardia

Very similar to supraventricular tachycardia, the difference being that the P waves are identifiable, so a more accurate identification than supraventricular tachycardia can be given. Both the effect and the treatment will be the same (if the rate is very rapid).

Supraventricular/ narrow complex tachycardia

Description

The impulses originate from somewhere within the atria (including the S-A node and A-V node). Because of the rapid ventricular rate (>150/min) P waves cannot be identified so neither can the exact origin of the impulse. This term is therefore used as a blanket term when the rhythm originates above the ventricles (supraventricular) and because of the rapid rate it is difficult or impossible to identify the rhythm accurately (figure 16). Alternatively the term 'narrow complex tachycardia' may be used, utilising the description of rate and the fact that the QRS is narrow (<0.12 sec). Either term may be used to describe the rhythm.

The arrhythmia may appear as paroxysms that start and end suddenly.

ECG characteristics

- Rate: 150–250/min
- Rhythm: regular
- P waves: cannot be identified
- P–R interval: cannot be identified
- QRS complex: normal, but occasionally an abnormality in the conduction of the impulse down the bundle branches (bundle branch block) may widen the QRS complex and it may then be difficult to differentiate between supraventricular tachycardia and ventricular tachycardia

Clinical significance

May occur for no apparent reason or may be due to damage to the S-A node, atria or A-V node (because of ischaemic heart disease). May also be caused by drug excess or sympathetic overactivity.

The very rapid rate will result in a lowering of cardiac output, with accompanying hypotension, poor tissue perfusion and cerebral hypoxia. The patient may complain of chest pain as the rapid rate may result in myocardial ischaemia.

Treatment

Oxygen therapy and analgesia may be required to treat the patient's presenting symptoms. Reflex vagal stimulation can be used (for example, carotid sinus massage or Valsalva's manoeuvre), in conjunction with monitoring of ECG and pulse. Adenosine 6 mg i.v. may be used to reduce the rate (can be repeated, if necessary at 12 mg), or if unsuccessful other antidysrhythmics may be used, or cardioversion (especially if the cardiac output is very low). Refer to current Resuscitation Council (UK) guidelines on the management of Narrow Complex Tachycardia.

Figure 16. Supraventricular (narrow complex) tachycardia

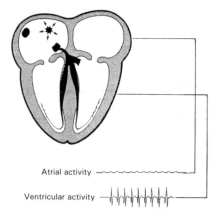

Atrial activity

Ventricular activity

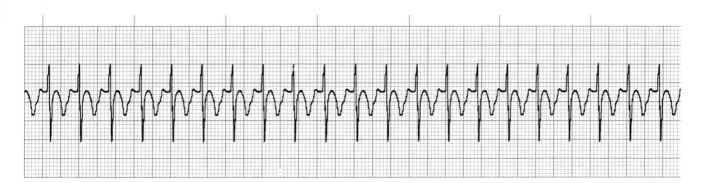

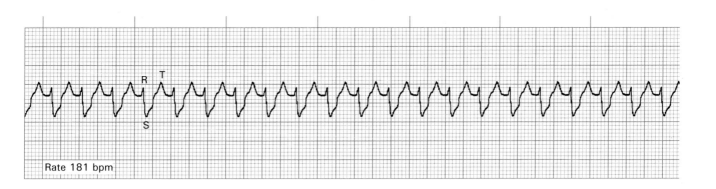

Rate 181 bpm

Ventricular dysrhythmias

Premature ventricular contractions (ventricular ectopics)

Description

The impulse originates somewhere within the ventricular myocardium. It is a premature beat arriving before the next normal beat is due and is followed by a compensatory pause. The QRS complex is wide and bizarre-looking (greater than 0.12 sec in duration) and the T wave is usually in the opposite direction to the QRS complex. The ectopic beat may just appear singly in an otherwise normal rhythm (figure 17).

ECG characteristics

- Rate: normal
- Rhythm: regular except for ventricular ectopics
- P waves: not seen
- P–R interval: not identifiable
- QRS complex: wide and bizarre (greater than 0.12 sec – three small squares)

Clinical significance

May be caused by damage to the ventricles (ischaemic heart disease), increased sympathetic or parasympathetic activity, hypoxia, acidosis, congestive cardiac failure or an affect of drug overdose.

Isolated ventricular ectopics may not be significant, but more frequent ventricular ectopics may result in a slight reduction in cardiac output, or may be the precursor of more serious ventricular dysrhythmias.

Treatment

May solely be observation and other appropriate management of ischaemic heart disease, if this may have caused the ectopics, but if the ventricular ectopics are very frequent and lead to a lowering in cardiac output they may require treatment, see Ventricular Tachycardia.

Figure 17. Premature ventricular contraction

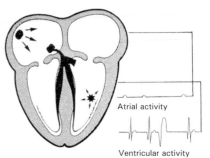

Atrial activity

Ventricular activity

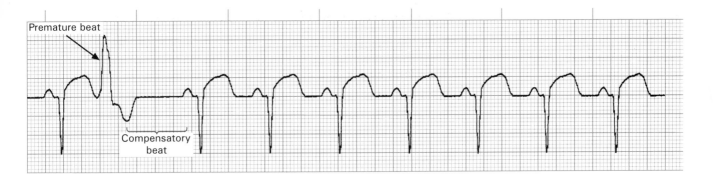

Premature beat

Compensatory
beat

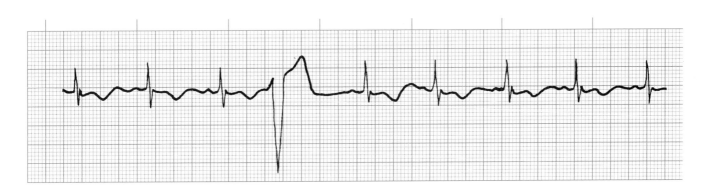

31

R-on-T ectopics

Description

The impulse originates somewhere in the ventricular myocardium, the same as ventricular ectopics (VEs). But with this type of VE the impulse is initiated earlier still so that the R wave of the VE coincides with the T wave of the previous beat (depolarization starts to occur while repolarization is still occurring) (figure 18).

ECG characteristics

- Rate: normal
- Rhythm: regular, except for the VEs
- P waves: not seen
- P–R interval: not identifiable
- QRS complex: wide and bizarre

(greater than 0.12 sec), with the R wave of the VE apparently running off the T wave of the previous beat

Clinical significance

The same as for VEs but with a greater risk of more serious ventricular dysrhythmias. Because depolarization starts again while repolarization is still occurring there is an increased risk of ventricular fibrillation.

Treatment

Close observation and management of the underlying cause of the VEs, if known, antidysrhythmics may be considered (see ventricular tachycardia page 34).

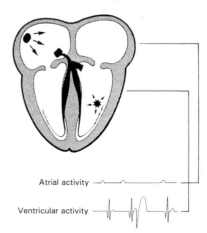

Figure 18. R-on-T ectopic

Atrial activity

Ventricular activity

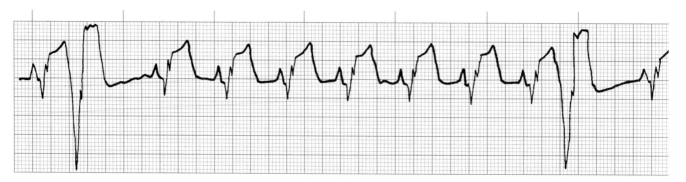

Ventricular bigeminy

In ventricular bigeminy every other beat is a ventricular ectopic, alternating with a normal beat. The interval between the normal beat and the ventricular ectopic is usually constant (figure 19).

Figure 19. Ventricular bigeminy

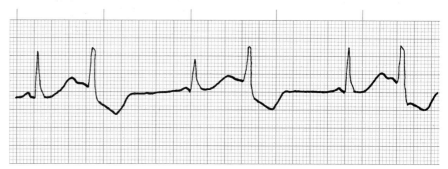

Ventricular trigeminy

Either every third beat is a ventricular ectopic or each normal beat is followed by two ventricular ectopics (figure 20).

Figure 20. Ventricular trigeminy

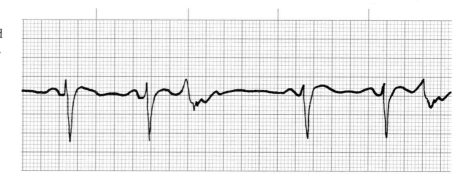

Ventricular/broad complex tachycardia

Description

Impulses originate from within the ventricular myocardium, appearing as three or more ventricular ectopics in a row. The ectopic foci may fire off at a rate of more than 150 bpm. It may be difficult to distinguish between ventricular (broad complex) tachycardia and supraventricular (narrow complex) tachycardia with an aberrant conduction. However, ventricular tachycardia is slightly irregular while supraventricular tachycardia is regular (figure 21). If the QRS is wide and the patient is compromised, treat as ventricular tachycardia, not supraventricular.

ECG characteristics

- Rate: more than 150 bpm
- Rhythm: slightly irregular
- P waves: usually present but may be buried in the QRS complex
- P–R interval: unidentifiable, the atria and ventricles are dissociated from each other
- QRS complex: wide and bizarre (greater than 0.12 sec)

Clinical significance

The rhythm may be caused by damage to the conduction pathway or ventricles (ischaemic heart disease), increased sympathetic or parasympathetic tone, hypoxia, acidosis, low serum potassium or affect of drug overdose.

If the rate is in excess of 150 bpm the cardiac output may be significantly affected resulting in a drop in both tissue perfusion and blood pressure. The signs and symptoms noted would be those of poor tissue perfusion and hypotension, and the rapid heart rate may be associated with myocardial ischaemia (angina) and pump failure. The dysrhythmia itself can be extremely dangerous resulting in unconsciousness and even death. Ventricular tachycardia may be a precursor of ventricular fibrillation.

Treatment

If the patient has no cardiac output, treat as for ventricular fibrillation.

If the patient has a cardiac output and has:
(1) A systolic blood pressure of greater than 90 mm Hg.
(2) A heart rate of less than 150 bpm.
(3) No evidence of heart failure.
(4) No evidence of chest pain.
The treatment should be based on the use of Amiodarone or Lignocaine; see the current Resuscitation Council (UK) guidelines on the management of Broad Complex Tachycardia.

If the patient has a cardiac output and has:
(1) A systolic blood pressure of less than 90 mm Hg.
(2) A heart rate of more than 150 bpm.
(3) Evidence of heart failure.
(4) Evidence of chest pain.

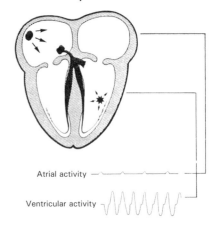

Figure 21. Ventricular (broad complex) tachycardia

Atrial activity

Ventricular activity

Seek expert help and consider the need
for urgent cardioversion, see the
current Resuscitation Council (UK)
guidelines on the management of
Broad Complex Tachycardia.

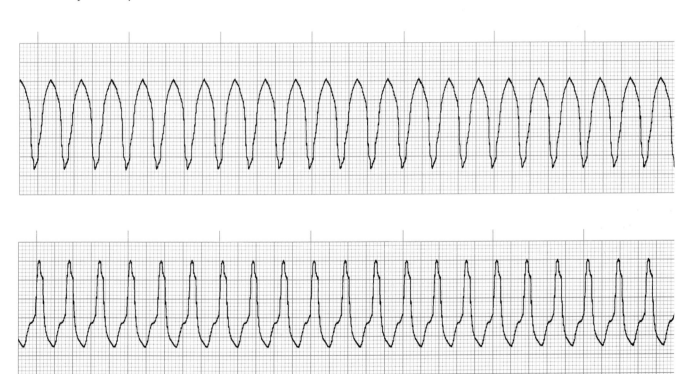

Ventricular fibrillation

Description

Impulses originate in one or more foci within the ventricles at a very fast rate, resulting in an uncoordinated activity within the ventricular myocardium (figure 22) and total loss of function of the ventricles.

ECG characteristics

- Rate: difficult to ascertain, fibrillation waves are seen at a rate in excess of 300/min
- Rhythm: irregular, uncoordinated and 'chaotic'
- P waves: may or may not be present, but are unrecognisable
- P–R interval: absent
- QRS complex: absent. The ectopic foci result in waves of fibrillation of varying amplitude and shape. The waves are known as coarse or fine depending upon amplitude

Clinical significance

May have the same causes as the other ventricular dysrhythmias. Ventricular fibrillation will result in a total loss of cardiac output.

Treatment

See the management of cardiac arrest, page 52.

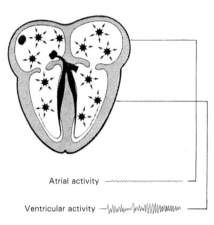

Figure 22(a). Ventricular fibrillation

Atrial activity

Ventricular activity

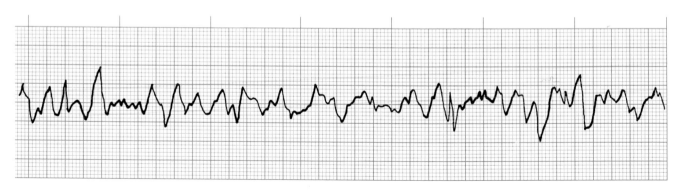

Figure 22(b). Ventricular fibrillation (coarse fine)

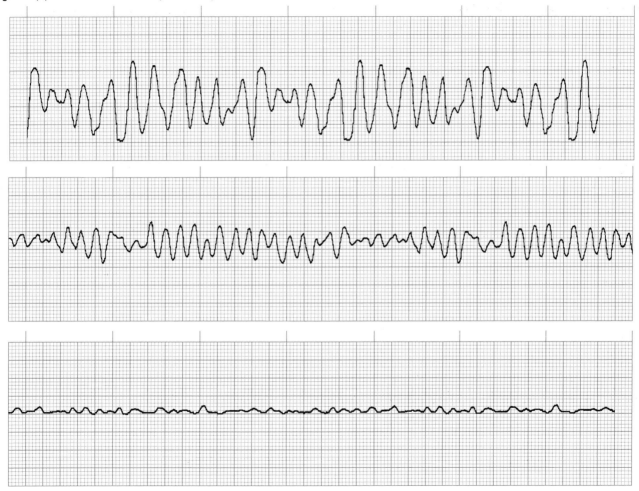

Ventricular standstill

Description

Total absence of ventricular activity. Only atrial activity is seen (figure 23), also known as P wave asystole.

ECG characteristics

Rate: ventricular – nil. Atrial rate may be normal
Rhythm: absent
P waves: normal
P–R interval: not identifiable
QRS complex: absent

Clinical significance

Results in an absence of cardiac output.

Treatment

See the management of cardiac arrest, page 52.

Figure 23. Ventricular standstill

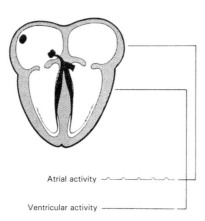

Atrial activity

Ventricular activity

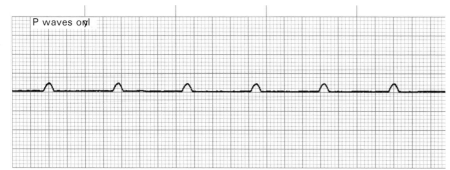

P waves only

Ventricular flutter

This term may be used to describe a form of ventricular fibrillation that is seen as a series of large wave-like oscillations (figure 24).

Figure 24.

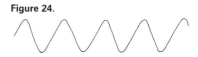

Asystole

There is a total absence of myocardial activity resulting in a loss of cardiac output (figure 25). Occasionally some bizarre looking movement may be noted on the trace, at an extremely slow rate, often called *agonal rhythm*, *post-mortem artefact* or *dying heart syndrome*.

Otherwise, all that can be seen is slight movement around the isoelectric line, rarely is it a straight line and if that is seen the patient must be checked, along with the ECG electrodes and equipment. For treatment see the management of cardiac arrest, page 52.

Figure 25.

Heart block

When a conduction defect exists, impulses may be delayed in their passage through the heart or even be totally prevented from passing to the ventricles. This is called heart block and it can be divided into several types.

First-degree heart block

Description

Here the impulse originates as normal in the S–A node but the conduction through the A–V node is slowed beyond normal limits, resulting in a longer than normal P–R interval. The rest of the complex is normal (figure 26).

ECG characteristics

- Rate: normal
- Rhythm: regular
- P waves: normal
- P–R interval: greater than 0.2 seç
- QRS complex: normal

Clinical significance

It may be caused by damage to the A–V node (as a result of organic heart disease), increased parasympathetic tone on the A–V node, hypoxia or the effect of some drugs. If the rate is normal there may be no adverse effect on the patient. The rhythm need only be noted because of an abnormally slow rate.

Treatment

No treatment is indicated if the rate is normal (if excessively slow, compromising the patient, it may be treated as sinus bradycardia, page 8). If, however, it is associated with organic heart disease (myocardial infarction, for example) the patient should be observed as the rhythm may progress to second- or third-degree heart block.

Figure 26. First-degree heart block

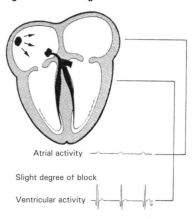

Atrial activity

Slight degree of block

Ventricular activity

(First-degree heart block)

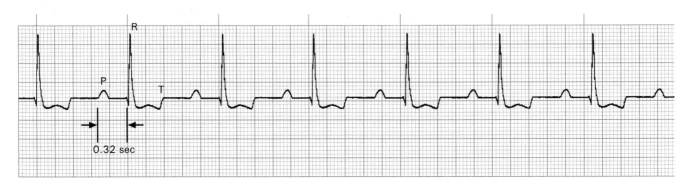

Second-degree heart block

This is further subdivided into:
(1) Mobitz type I (Wenckebach phenomenon)
(2) Mobitz type II

Mobitz type I (Wenckebach phenomenon)

Description

The impulse originates in the S–A node as normal, but the conduction through the A–V node is abnormal. The impulse is delayed slightly longer each time it passes through the A–V node. This results in an increasing P–R interval until eventually one impulse from the S–A node is completely blocked while the impulse following is allowed to pass through the A–V node at a more normal interval. This is seen on the ECG as an increasing P–R interval until a P wave is seen that is not followed by a QRS complex. This is usually seen as a cycle with one more P wave in the cycle than QRS complexes (although the number of complexes in each cycle may occasionally vary) (figure 27).

ECG characteristics

- Rate: normal or slow
- Rhythm: P waves regular; QRS complexes irregular
- P waves: normal
- P–R interval: increasing in length. May be normal at the beginning of the cycle.
- QRS complex: normal

Clinical significance

May be caused for the same reasons as first-degree heart block. If the rate is normal there may be little or no adverse effect on the patient. If the rate is excessively slow cardiac output may deteriorate, resulting in the signs and symptoms of low cardiac output.

Treatment

If the cardiac output is normal, no treatment is required, although the rhythm does carry the risk of deterioration to complete heart block. If the patient exhibits the signs and symptoms of a compromised cardiac output, a reduction in blood pressure, increased peripheral vasoconstriction, poor tissue perfusion, confusion and even unconsciousness, he will require oxygen to relieve the hypoxia. The slow rate and compromised circulation will require treatment with Atropine, as it increases the rate at the S–A node and therefore the ventricular rate (see

treatment of Sinus Bradycardia).
External pacing or an Adrenaline
infusion may be required if the
atropine does not help.

Figure 27. Mobitz type I (Wenckebach phenomenon)

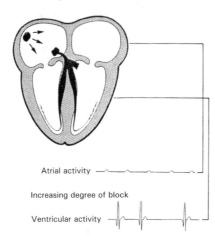

Atrial activity

Increasing degree of block

Ventricular activity

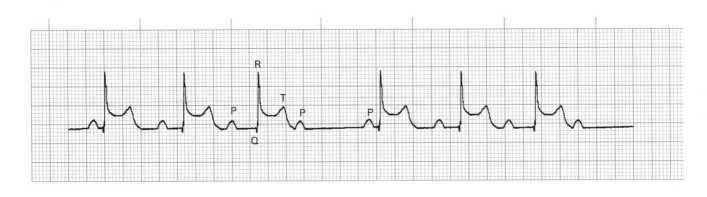

Mobitz type II

Description

Very similar to Mobitz type I, the difference being that the A–V node blocks a regular number of impulses allowing every second, third or fourth, etc. impulse through to the ventricles. The rate of block is usually regular, but may be irregular. The individual rhythm may be described as a 2:1, 3:1, 4:1, etc. block depending upon how many P waves are noted prior to each QRS complex (figure 28).

ECG characteristics

▓ Rate: normal or slow
▓ Rhythm: P waves regular, QRS complexes regular (occasionally irregular)
▓ P waves: normal
▓ P–R interval: When seen it may be normal or prolonged but is constant. There may be two, three or more P waves prior to each QRS complex.
▓ QRS complex: normal or occasionally widened

Clinical significance

The same as Mobitz type I.

Treatment

As for Mobitz type I.

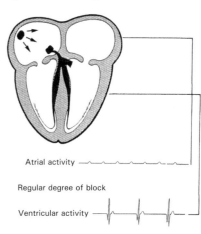

Figure 28. Mobitz type II

Atrial activity

Regular degree of block

Ventricular activity

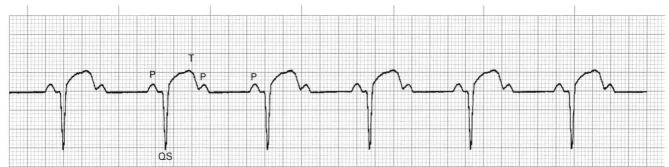

43

Third-degree heart block

This is also known as complete heart block or complete atrioventricular dissociation.

Description

The A–V node does not conduct any impulses and therefore the atria and ventricles beat completely independently of each other. The S–A node continues to pace the atria but because the impulses are not conducted through the A–V node an ectopic focus in the ventricles takes over the control of the ventricles. If the ectopic focus is high up in the ventricles near the bundle of His the QRS complexes may appear quite normal. If the ectopic focus is low in the ventricles the QRS complex will appear wide and bizarre. The P waves and QRS complexes have no relationship to each other, and the P waves are often lost in the QRS complexes. Occasionally a P wave may be seen prior to the QRS complex, but this is purely a coincidence, and the two have no relationship to each other, and are completely dissociated (figure 29).

ECG characteristics

- Rate: atrial rate may be normal, ventricular rate may be 20–50 bpm
- Rhythm: atria regular, ventricles usually regular
- P waves: normal, but may not be seen as they may be buried in the QRS complexes
- P–R interval: variable, when seen
- QRS complex: abnormal, the width and shape may vary depending upon exact focus

Clinical significance

The rhythm may be caused by damage to the A–V node, bundle of His or bundle branches (as in ischaemic heart disease or trauma) or increased parasympathetic tone. The ventricular rate is usually slow with its associated reduction in cardiac output. The patient, therefore, will show the signs and symptoms of a compromised cardiac output, because of the slow rate ventricular dysrhythmias may appear, and there is also the risk of deterioration to ventricular standstill.

Treatment

If the rate is sufficient to maintain cardiac output little treatment may be required. However, if the patient shows the signs and symptoms of the reduced cardiac output, supportive therapy will be required. Treatment will be that of a bradycardia resulting in a compromised cardiac output (see Sinus Bradycardia) and may include external pacing, prior to temporary transvenous pacing. If necessary followed later by a permanent pacemaker.

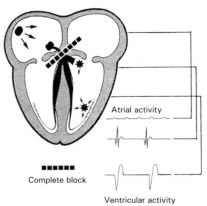

Figure 29. Third-degree heart block (complete heart block)

Atrial activity

Complete block

Ventricular activity

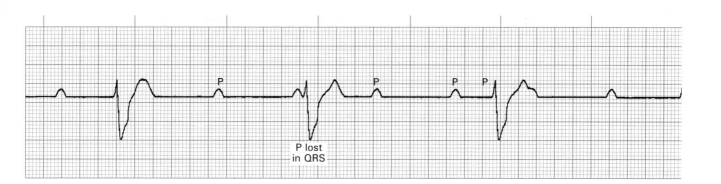

P lost
in QRS

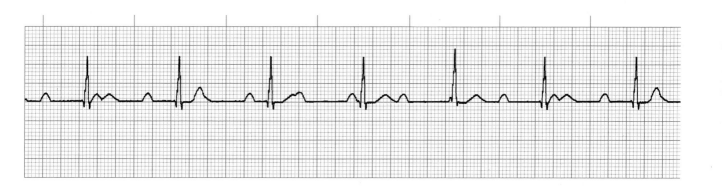

45

Stokes–Adams attack

Description

The underlying rhythm may be regular and relatively normal, or there may be some degree of heart block. There is a sudden loss of cardiac output resulting in the associated signs and symptoms. The rhythm causing this is often ventricular standstill (P wave asystole), but may occasionally be asystole or even an episode of ventricular fibrillation.

The rhythm may revert spontaneously or may require the specific treatment of the presenting rhythm to enable the resumption of a more normal rhythm and cardiac output (figure 30).

ECG characteristics

- Rate: during attack – nil
- Rhythm: may or may not be normal, during attack will be absent.
- P waves: may or may not be present
- P–R interval: absent
- QRS complex: absent during the attack

Clinical significance

The dysrhythmia may be caused by any of the reasons that may cause heart block.

The sudden total loss of cardiac output produces a dizzy episode (within 5 sec), loss of consciousness (after 10 sec), fits (after 15 sec) and signs of cardiac arrest after 30 sec. If the patient does not revert spontaneously death will ensue unless resuscitation is attempted.

Occasionally if the patient is upright when the Stokes–Adams attack occurs the jolt as he hits the ground may revert the dysrhythmia and he may appear to have just fainted.

Treatment

If the patient reverts spontaneously, general observation may be all that is required (including monitor observation). Oxygen therapy will be required if the patient is hypoxic. If he does not revert spontaneously he will show the signs and symptoms of cardiac arrest (see section on cardiac arrest, page 52).

Figure 30. Stokes–Adams attack

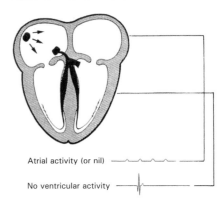

Atrial activity (or nil)

No ventricular activity

May revert spontaneously

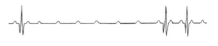

OR

OR

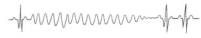

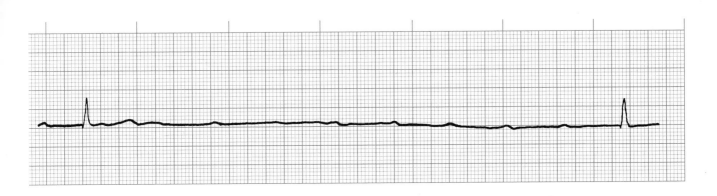

47

Paced beats

Description

Because the underlying rhythm is abnormal and very slow, a temporary transvenous or permanent internal electrical pacemaker is used to increase the ventricular rate. The end of the pacing catheter is lodged in the apex of the right ventricle. The P waves and paced beats may or may not appear dissociated from each other. Though the QRS complex seen appears wide and bizarre it results in a good ventricular output (figure 31). An upright faint line may be noted at the start of the QRS complex, this is the pacing artefact caused by the pacing stimulus.

ECG characteristics

- Rate: ventricular rate normal (70–80 bpm)
- Rhythm: regular
- P waves: may or may not be noted
- P–R interval: absent
- QRS complex: wide and bizarre

Clinical significance

The treatment of a dysrhythmia (complete heart block), therefore, will result in an improvement in the patient's condition and satisfactory cardiac output.

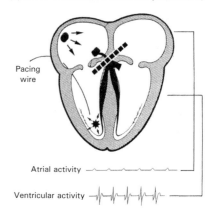

Figure 31. Paced beats (internal pacemaker)

Pacing wire

Atrial activity

Ventricular activity

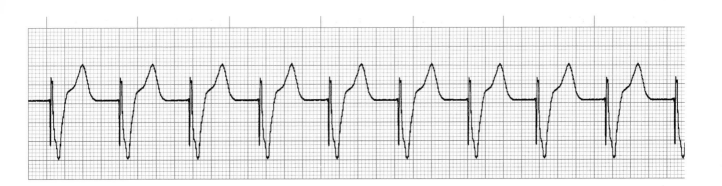

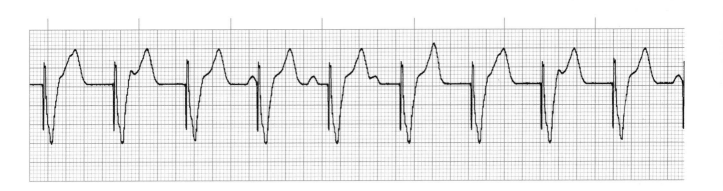

49

Bundle branch block

This occurs when there is damage to one of the branches of the bundle of His, and results in an abnormal conduction of the impulse through the bundle branches. This may be seen on the QRS complex as a notch, the position of the notch varying according to the position of the block. A 12-lead ECG is needed to diagnose whether right or left bundle branch block is present.

The bundle branch block may be of little significance, or may be the precursor of a total block at the bundle of His.

It is important to note on the monitor that this is recognised as an addition to an underlying rhythm. For example, a notch on the QRS complex but no P wave would be suggestive of a mid-nodal rhythm, but if the notch is seen and a P wave is noted prior to the complex then a bundle branch block may be seen (figure 32). The distortion to the QRS complex may also widen the complex, resulting in a narrow complex tachycardia appearing as a broad complex tachycardia (see ventricular tachycardia).

Figure 32.

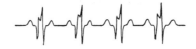

Signs of myocardial ischaemia, injury and infarction

It is important to remember that to accurately diagnose myocardial ischaemia, injury or infarction on the ECG, a 12-lead ECG must be recorded. Occasionally the signs may be seen on a monitoring lead, but as these signs can only be *suggestive* of ischaemia, injury or infarction they are not conclusive or diagnostic. However, these changes may result in an apparent distortion of the QRS complex.

If an area of the myocardium is dead as a result of myocardial infarction the myocardial cells cannot be polarized or depolarized, so if an electrode is placed over this area it will only pick up the electrical activity opposite (as if looking through a 'window').

If an area of myocardium is ischaemic or injured then abnormalities of the T wave and S–T segment may be seen on an electrode placed over this area.

Ischaemia: May be seen as an inverted T wave.

Injury:　This is seen as a raised S–T segment, usually the higher the S–T segment the greater the degree of injury.

Infarction: This is seen as a deep Q wave (greater than a third the depth of the total height/depth of the QRS complex), in combination with the signs of ischaemia and injury.

Around an area of infarction is an area of injury which in turn is surrounded by an area of ischaemia (see figure 33).

If the electrode used is placed on the opposite side of the infarction, injury or ischaemia, the opposite or reciprocal effect will be seen on the ECG.

Figure 33. Signs of myocardial ischaemia, injury and infarction on the ECG

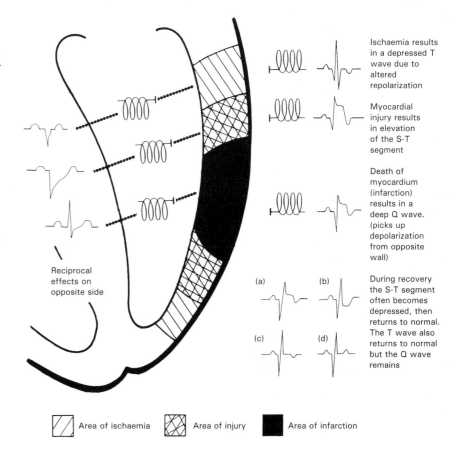

Reciprocal effects on opposite side

Ischaemia results in a depressed T wave due to altered repolarization

Myocardial injury results in elevation of the S-T segment

Death of myocardium (infarction) results in a deep Q wave. (picks up depolarization from opposite wall)

(a)　(b)

(c)　(d)

During recovery the S-T segment often becomes depressed, then returns to normal. The T wave also returns to normal but the Q wave remains

▨ Area of ischaemia　　▩ Area of injury　　■ Area of infarction

51

Cardiac arrest

By definition, cardiac arrest is a failure of the heart to maintain an adequate cerebral circulation, in the absence of a causative or irreversible disease. This tells us that cardiac arrest is a potentially reversible situation while death, of course, is not.

Although there may be many causes of cardiac arrest, both the effect on the patient and the treatment are the same.

Effect on the patient

If the circulation stops, and therefore the blood flow to the brain ceases, the partial pressure of oxygen (PO_2) in the cerebral vessels will drop to 20 mmHg within 10 sec causing loss of consciousness. The cerebral PO_2 drops to zero within approximately 1 min causing respiration to cease. Within minutes of this occurrence there is irreversible brain damage. As the blood flow to the tissues has ceased there is a general tissue hypoxia and a build-up of waste products, as they cannot be removed. All these effects lead to a number of signs that may be used to assist the diagnosis of cardiac arrest. But there are two signs that will always be present and these two alone are all that are required to diagnose cardiac arrest.

Diagnosis

The two signs that are required are:
(1) loss of consciousness,
(2) loss of central pulses (carotid, femoral).
If these signs are present the patient is in a state of cardiac arrest. Other signs develop as the general tissue and cerebral hypoxia increase, and there is irreversible brain damage.

Cerebral signs

Respiration ceases (similarly respiratory arrest leads to cardiac arrest if untreated); pupils dilate and become unresponsive.

General signs

There is pallor or greyness (other colours may be seen depending upon cause of arrest, such as the cherry red colour of carbon monoxide poisoning); cyanosis, central and/or peripheral; cold, clammy skin.

Treatment

The management consists of addressing three main areas:
(1) Airway: must be cleared and secured,
(2) Breathing: adequate ventilation must be initiated/achieved and include high flow oxygen,
(3) Circulation: imitate/support with external chest compression.

Airway

This may be opened by the use of head tilt/chin lift or jaw thrust, cleared, if necessary, with suction and maintained by good positioning. The use of basic airway adjuncts (oral or nasal airway, Laryngeal Mask airway or similar) may aid airway management, the airway will only be secure following endotracheal intubation.

Breathing

Support of ventilation must result in oxygen effectively entering the lungs. This may be by expired air resuscitation, via an appropriate aid, initially. The patient should be ventilated via a suitable Bag-Valve-Mask (BVM) with high flow oxygen as a standard. Once the airway is secure ventilation will continue with bag to endotracheal tube or mechanical ventilator to endotracheal tube.

Circulation

If the patient's collapse is witnessed and cardiac arrest is confirmed, a precordial 'thump' should be used. This may result in a return of cardiac output; therefore a central pulse must be palpated after this action. If cardiac arrest continues effective external chest compression (ECC) must be implemented.

Effective ventilation and ECC must be continued throughout resuscitation attempts. Both effectiveness and safety of the ECC must be confirmed. The efficiency of ECC can be checked by palpating the carotid or femoral pulse, a pulse should be felt with each compression. Ensure that the operators shoulders are directly above the patient's chest, that the operator is in a position such that ECC is delivered with straight arms (locked elbows), that the rate of ECC and depth of the compressions meet with current Resuscitation Council (UK) guidelines. At the earliest opportunity, without compromising the basic management, an ECG monitor should be attached to the patient, to allow assessment of the rhythm. While the monitor is observed there must be a pause in ECC, as ECC will cause an artefact on the monitor, this pause should be for the minimum period to confirm the rhythm to be managed and should not exceed 10 seconds. The only other times that there is a pause in ECC, or it is stopped, is during defibrillation, on return of cardiac output, or when resuscitation is abandoned.

Defibrillation

If the patient is in a shockable rhythm – ventricular fibrillation (VF) or pulseless ventricular tachycardia (VT), defibrillation is required. Individual defibrillators may vary slightly in their layout, make yourself familiar with the defibrillator you will use.

The preferred method of defibrillation is via adhesive pads – hands free technique. Alternatively hand held paddles will need to be held on the patient's chest. If using hand held paddles, electrode gel pads must be placed between the paddles and the skin.

The adhesive pads should be applied firmly to the patient's chest: one immediately below the right clavicle to the right of the sternum. The second on the lower left chest, located between a line from the centre of the left clavicle and a line in the centre of the axilla, with the bottom edge of the pad immediately above the bottom edge of the ribs. Hand held paddles must be held in the same position. The monitor should be checked immediately prior to defibrillation to ensure that the patient is still in the rhythm to be defibrillated.

During defibrillation ensure that no one is in contact with the patient, or anything conductive that the patient is in contact with. (Ensure that appropriate training is undertaken prior to attempting to use a defibrillator.)

Defibrillation should be repeated according to current guidelines, ECC might need to be recommenced immediately after defibrillation if there is still no cardiac output, followed by further defibrillation if the patient is still in VF/VT.

Energy levels for defibrillation should be administered following current Resuscitation Council (UK) guidelines and may vary dependent upon whether monophasic or biphasic equipment is used.

Figure 34. Arrythmias that may be seen prior to or during a cardiac arrest

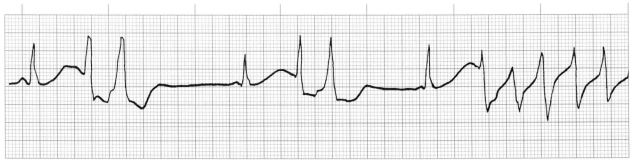

Ventricular trigeminy ⟶ Ventricular tachycardia

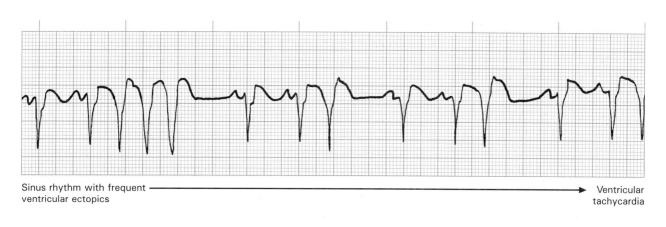

Sinus rhythm with frequent ──────────────────────────────► Ventricular
ventricular ectopics   tachycardia

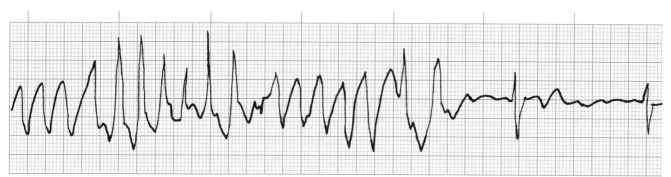

Spontaneous reversion of ventricular fibrillation
to a more normal rhythm

Drugs used in the management of adult cardiac arrest

Oxygen

High flow oxygen is required throughout the resuscitation process.

Adrenaline

1 mg intravenously (double dose via ET tube). Administered during periods of ECC, at intervals of 3 minutes. Its prime use is to aid the effectiveness of ECC.

Atropine

3 mg intravenously (double dose via ET tube). Following the initial administration of adrenaline, in the management of asystole or pulseless electrical activity with a rate of less than 60 bpm.

Amiodarone

300 mg intravenously. Following the administration of adrenaline in the management of Ventricular Fibrillation resistant to defibrillation (after first sequence of defibrillation).

Success or?

Successful resuscitation is indicated by a return of cardiac output, which is maintained beyond the effects of the adrenaline administered during the resuscitation attempt. Dependent upon the cause of arrest, its duration and the effects of hypoxia, on the patient, respiratory effort may return or still require support. Equally level of consciousness will vary.

If the patient fails to respond to resuscitation efforts, there is no return of spontaneous circulation in spite of appropriate management (according to current Resuscitation Council (UK) guidelines). Continue effective ventilation and ECC, along with appropriate advanced management until the resuscitation attempt is no longer in the patient's interests and a decision to abandon resuscitation is made.

Aftercare

When the patient has a return of spontaneous circulation, during the recovery period, the following steps should be undertaken:

(1) Maintain the airway management.
(2) Assess the patient's consciousness level, heart rate, respiratory rate, ECG rhythm, etc.
(3) Assess blood gases and support the patient's respiratory state.
(4) Assess the 12 lead ECG and appropriate blood results, and initiate other supportive treatment as required.
(5) Initiate any required supportive management in ITU, including management of any cause of unconsciousness.
(6) Check for injuries incurred as a result of resuscitation or during the initial collapse and treat as necessary. (For example, fractured ribs, flail segment, pneumothorax, head injury, etc.).
(7) Discover why the patient had a cardiac arrest. Observe him – he may do it again!
(8) Consider other post-resuscitation management, including thrombolysis.
(9) If the patient is conscious and distressed reassure him. Suitable analgesia and/or sedation may be required.

Index

The
ECG-
What does it tell?

Jim Gardiner

RGN, RNT, Cert. Ed(FE), ALS(I), EPLS(I)
Resuscitation Officer, Hereford Hospitals NHS Trust

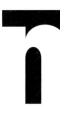

First published in 1981 by:
Stanley Thornes (Publishers) Ltd

This edition published in 2005 by:
Nelson Thornes Ltd
Delta Place
27 Bath Road
CHELTENHAM
GL53 7TH
United Kingdom

05 06 07 08 09 / 10 9 8 7 6 5 4 3 2 1

A catalogue record for this book is available from the British Library

ISBN 0 7487 8523 X

Illustrations by Acorn Bookwork and Wearset
Page make-up by Acorn Bookwork

Printed in Croatia by Zrinski